Cin,
Hope you like!
I bought one
too - will jam
together. ♥

5-2020

MW00425356

the Purpose of Journaling

Cancer. It is a word that causes fear to grip your heart and mind.

The experience of hearing this word in the same sentence as my Dad was something I wasn't prepared for emotionally. Our family was devastated and overwhelmed with the news, just as so many families know all to well.

I will never forget hearing someone say to me when I shared this news with them, "Cancer isn't always a death sentence."

One of the most important things about the fight against cancer is keeping your mind positive through the process, whether it is you or a loved one.

Knowing the importance of keeping your reflections positive, I created this journal for my own family and others, like us, who are facing cancer.

How to use this journal

Meditate on the Bible verses and quote for each day of the next 31 days.

Positive Reflection is the area where you jot down anything that makes you think positive. You can use these space to write your thoughts on the verse or quote for the day.

Releasing Negativity is the area that you write down anything that is causing you negative thoughts. Release them in writing and leave them there.

Words of Encouragement is the area where you record any encouragement that came your way that day, whether it is from your own thoughts or words of others.

I'm Thankful for is the area where you count your blessings because even on the hardest of days, there is something to be thankful for each day.

Day One

"Death and life are in the power of the tongue: and they that love it should eat the fruit thereof."

Proverbs 18:21

Positive Reflection: _____
_____
_____
_____
_____
_____

Releasing Negativity: _____
_____
_____
_____
_____
_____

"The greatest healing therapy is friendship and love."

Hubert H. Humphrey

Words of Encouragement: _____

_____

_____

_____

_____

_____

_____

I'm Thankful for: _____

_____

_____

_____

_____

_____

_____

Day Two

"So do not fear, for I am with you; do not be dismayed, for I am your God. I will strengthen you and help you; I will uphold you with my righteous right hand."

Isaiah 41:10

Positive Reflection: _____

_____

_____

_____

_____

_____

Releasing Negativity: _____

_____

_____

_____

_____

_____

"love one another and help others to rise to the higher levels, simply by pouring out love. love is infectious and the greatest healing energy."

Sai Baba

Words of Encouragement: ───────────────

─────────────────────────────────

─────────────────────────────────

─────────────────────────────────

─────────────────────────────────

─────────────────────────────────

─────────────────────────────────

I'm Thankful for: ───────────────

─────────────────────────────────

─────────────────────────────────

─────────────────────────────────

─────────────────────────────────

─────────────────────────────────

─────────────────────────────────

─────────────────────────────────

Day three

"Truly he is my rock and my salvation; he is my fortress.
I will not be shaken. My salvation and my honor
depend on God; he is my mighty rock, my refuge. Trust
in him at all times, you people; pour out your hearts
to him, for God is our refuge."

Psalms 62:6-8

Positive Reflection: _____

_____

_____

_____

_____

_____

Releasing Negativity: _____

_____

_____

_____

_____

_____

"Healing is a matter
of time, but it is
sometimes also a matter
of opportunity."
Hippocrates

Words of Encouragement: ——————————————————

——————————————————————————————————————

——————————————————————————————————————

——————————————————————————————————————

——————————————————————————————————————

——————————————————————————————————————

——————————————————————————————————————

I'm Thankful for: ———————————————————————

——————————————————————————————————————

——————————————————————————————————————

——————————————————————————————————————

——————————————————————————————————————

——————————————————————————————————————

——————————————————————————————————————

Day Four

"And even the very hairs of your head are all numbered. So don't be afraid; you are worth more than many sparrows."

Matthew 10:30-31

Positive Reflection: _____

_____

_____

_____

_____

_____

Releasing Negativity: _____

_____

_____

_____

_____

_____

"The friend who can be silent with us
in a moment of despair or confusion,
who can stay with us in an hour
of grief and bereavement, who can
tolerate not knowing... not healing, not
curing... that is a friend who cares."

Henri Nouwen

Words of Encouragement: _____

_____

_____

_____

_____

_____

_____

I'm Thankful for: _____

_____

_____

_____

_____

_____

_____

Day Five

"Cast all your anxiety on him because he cares for you."

1 Peter 5:7

Positive Reflection: _____

_____

_____

_____

_____

_____

_____

Releasing Negativity: _____

_____

_____

_____

_____

_____

_____

"The wish for healing
has always been
half of health."
Lucius Annaeus Seneca

Words of Encouragement: _____
_____
_____
_____
_____
_____
_____

I'm Thankful for: _____
_____
_____
_____
_____
_____
_____

Day Six

"A cheerful heart is good medicine, but a crushed spirit dries up the bones."

Proverbs 17:22

Positive Reflection: _____

_____

_____

_____

_____

_____

_____

Releasing Negativity: _____

_____

_____

_____

_____

_____

_____

"Laughter is important, not only because it makes us happy, it also has actual health benefits. And that's because laughter completely engages the body and releases the mind. It connects us to others, and that in itself has a healing effect."

Marlo Thomas

Words of Encouragement: ————————————

—————————————————————————
—————————————————————————
—————————————————————————
—————————————————————————
—————————————————————————
—————————————————————————

I'm Thankful for: ——————————————

—————————————————————————
—————————————————————————
—————————————————————————
—————————————————————————
—————————————————————————
—————————————————————————

Day Seven

"The lord will fight for you; you
need only to be still."

Exodus 14:14

Positive Reflection: _____

_____

_____

_____

_____

_____

Releasing Negativity: _____

_____

_____

_____

_____

_____

"Healing takes courage, and we all have courage, even if we have to dig a little to find it."

Tori Amos

Words of Encouragement: ─────────────

──────────────────────────────

──────────────────────────────

──────────────────────────────

──────────────────────────────

──────────────────────────────

──────────────────────────────

I'm Thankful for: ───────────────

──────────────────────────────

──────────────────────────────

──────────────────────────────

──────────────────────────────

──────────────────────────────

──────────────────────────────

Day Eight

"Then your light will break forth like the dawn, and your healing will quickly appear; then your righteousness will go before you, and the glory of the lord will be your rear guard. Then you will call, and the lord will answer; you will cry for help, and he will say: Here am I."

Isaiah 58:8-9

Positive Reflection: _____

_____

_____

_____

_____

_____

Releasing Negativity: _____

_____

_____

_____

_____

_____

"Part of the healing process is sharing with other people who care."

Jerry Cantrell

Words of Encouragement: _____

_____

_____

_____

_____

_____

_____

I'm Thankful for: _____

_____

_____

_____

_____

_____

_____

_____

Day Nine

"For I know the plans I have for you, declares the lord, plans to prosper you and not to harm you, plans to give you hope and a future."

Jeremiah 29:11

Positive Reflection: _____

_____

_____

_____

_____

_____

_____

Releasing Negativity: _____

_____

_____

_____

_____

_____

_____

"The words of kindness are more healing to a drooping heart than balm or honey."

Sarah Fielding

Words of Encouragement: _____

_____

_____

_____

_____

_____

I'm Thankful for: _____

_____

_____

_____

_____

_____

Day Ten

"Cast your cares on the lord and he will sustain you; he will never let the righteous be shaken."

Psalms 55:22

Positive Reflection: _____

_____

_____

_____

_____

_____

Releasing Negativity: _____

_____

_____

_____

_____

_____

"Natural forces within us are the true healers of disease."
Hippocrates

Words of Encouragement: _____

_____

_____

_____

_____

_____

_____

I'm Thankful for: _____

_____

_____

_____

_____

_____

_____

Day Eleven

"Have I not commanded you? Be strong and courageous. Do not be afraid; do not be discouraged, for the lord your God will be with you wherever you go."

Joshua 1:9

Positive Reflection: _____

_____

_____

_____

_____

_____

Releasing Negativity: _____

_____

_____

_____

_____

_____

"Of one thing I am certain, the body is not the measure of healing, peace is the measure."

Phyllis McGinley

Words of Encouragement: _____

_____

_____

_____

_____

_____

_____

I'm Thankful for: _____

_____

_____

_____

_____

_____

_____

Day Twelve

"But for you who revere my name, the sun of righteousness will rise with healing in its rays. And you will go out and frolic like well-fed calves."
Malachi 4:2

Positive Reflection: _____

_____

_____

_____

_____

_____

Releasing Negativity: _____

_____

_____

_____

_____

_____

"When it comes to my salvation, all I need is Jesus; after my salvation, everything is Jesus plus the church... When people preach that all you need is Jesus, they cut you and I off from one of the greatest sources of healing, which is the body of Christ. Don't go it alone - you won't make it."

Josh McDowell

Words of Encouragement: _____
_____
_____
_____
_____
_____

I'm Thankful for: _____
_____
_____
_____
_____
_____

Day Thirteen

" For everything that was written in the past was written to teach us, so that through the endurance taught in the Scriptures and the encouragement they provide we might have hope."

Romans 15:4

Positive Reflection: _____

_____

_____

_____

_____

_____

Releasing Negativity: _____

_____

_____

_____

_____

_____

"Trying to suppress or eradicate symptoms on the physical level can be extremely important, but there's more to healing than that: dealing with psychological, emotional and spiritual issues involved in treating sickness is equally important."
Marianne Williamson

Words of Encouragement: _____
_____
_____
_____
_____
_____

I'm Thankful for: _____
_____
_____
_____
_____
_____

Day Fourteen

"Praise the lord, my soul, and forget not all his benefits - who forgives all your sins and heals all your diseases, who redeems your life from the pit and crowns you with love and compassion."

Psalms 103:2-4

Positive Reflection: _____

_____

_____

_____

_____

_____

Releasing Negativity: _____

_____

_____

_____

_____

_____

"Nothing is so healing
as the human touch."
Bobby Fischer

Words of Encouragement: ——————————————
————————————————————————
————————————————————————
————————————————————————
————————————————————————
————————————————————————
————————————————————————

I'm Thankful for: ——————————————————
————————————————————————
————————————————————————
————————————————————————
————————————————————————
————————————————————————
————————————————————————

Day Fifteen

"And we know that in all things God works for the good of those who love him, who have been called according to his purpose."

Romans 8:28

Positive Reflection: _____

_____

_____

_____

_____

_____

_____

Releasing Negativity: _____

_____

_____

_____

_____

_____

_____

"If the brain expects that a treatment will work, it sends healing chemicals into the bloodstream, which facilitates that. And the opposite is equally true and equally powerful: When the brain expects that a therapy will not work, it doesn't. It's called the 'nocebo' effect."

Bruce Lipton

Words of Encouragement: _____

_____

_____

_____

_____

_____

_____

I'm Thankful for: _____

_____

_____

_____

_____

_____

_____

_____

Day Sixteen

"God is our refuge and strength, an ever-present help in trouble. Therefore we will not fear, though the earth give way and the mountains fall into the heart of the sea, though its waters roar and foam and the mountains quake with their surging."

Psalms 46:1-3

Positive Reflection: _____

_____

_____

_____

_____

_____

Releasing Negativity: _____

_____

_____

_____

_____

_____

"I make jokes because humor is the greatest healing factor that there is."

Dick Dale

Words of Encouragement: _____

_____

_____

_____

_____

_____

_____

I'm Thankful for: _____

_____

_____

_____

_____

_____

_____

Day Seventeen

"Now faith is confidence in what we hope for and assurance about what we do not see."

Hebrews 11:1

Positive Reflection: _____

_____

_____

_____

_____

_____

_____

Releasing Negativity: _____

_____

_____

_____

_____

_____

_____

"I don't know if I realized that I was funny, but I realized how healing and important humor was in my childhood."
Bonnie Hunt

Words of Encouragement: _____

_____

_____

_____

_____

_____

_____

I'm Thankful for: _____

_____

_____

_____

_____

_____

Day Eighteen

"Because you have so little faith. Truly I tell you, if you have faith as small as a mustard seed, you can say to this mountain, 'Move from here to there,' and it will move. Nothing will be impossible for you."

Matthew 17:20

Positive Reflection: _____

_____

_____

_____

_____

_____

Releasing Negativity: _____

_____

_____

_____

_____

_____

"It's interesting when you read the life of Christ how much of his time he spent healing the sick. There must have been a reason for that - he was modelling for us what it is we are intended to do by following his path."

Francis Collins

Words of Encouragement: _____
_____
_____
_____
_____
_____
_____

I'm Thankful for: _____
_____
_____
_____
_____
_____
_____

Day Nineteen

"...because you know that the testing of your faith produces perseverance."

James 1:3

Positive Reflection: _____

_____

_____

_____

_____

_____

Releasing Negativity: _____

_____

_____

_____

_____

_____

"The birth of the baby Jesus stands
as the most significant event in
all history, because it has meant
the pouring into a sick world the
healing medicine of love which has
transformed all manner of hearts
for almost two thousand years."
George Matthew Adams

Words of Encouragement: _____
_____
_____
_____
_____
_____
_____

I'm Thankful for: _____
_____
_____
_____
_____
_____
_____

Day Twenty

"And without faith it is impossible to please God, because anyone who comes to him must believe that he exists and that he rewards those who earnestly seek him."

Hebrews 11:6

Positive Reflection: _____

_____

_____

_____

_____

_____

Releasing Negativity: _____

_____

_____

_____

_____

_____

"Music is universal; it's healing."

Crystal Gayle

Words of Encouragement: —————————————————

_____

_____

_____

_____

_____

_____

I'm Thankful for: ———————————————————————

_____

_____

_____

_____

_____

_____

_____

Day Twenty-One

"Is anyone among you in trouble? Let them pray. Is anyone happy? Let them sing songs of praise. Is anyone among you sick? Let them call the elders of the church to pray over them and anoint them with oil in the name of the Lord."

James 5:13-14

Positive Reflection: _____

_____

_____

_____

_____

_____

Releasing Negativity: _____

_____

_____

_____

_____

_____

"Our greatest happiness does not
depend on the condition of life
in which chance has placed us,
but is always the result of a good
conscience, good health, occupation,
and freedom in all just pursuits."

Thomas Jefferson

Words of Encouragement: _____

_____

_____

_____

_____

_____

_____

I'm Thankful for: _____

_____

_____

_____

_____

_____

_____

Day Twenty-two

"Through him you believe in God, who raised him from the dead and glorified him, and so your faith and hope are in God."

1 Peter 1:21

Positive Reflection: _____
_____
_____
_____
_____
_____

Releasing Negativity: _____
_____
_____
_____
_____
_____

"The first wealth is health."

Ralph Waldo Emerson

Words of Encouragement: _____
_____
_____
_____
_____
_____
_____

I'm Thankful for: _____
_____
_____
_____
_____
_____
_____

Day Twenty-three

"Consequently, faith comes from hearing the message, and the message is heard through the word about Christ."

Romans 10:17

Positive Reflection: _____
_____
_____
_____
_____
_____

Releasing Negativity: _____
_____
_____
_____
_____
_____

"Sleep is that golden
chain that ties health
and our bodies together."
Thomas Dekker

Words of Encouragement: _____

_____

_____

_____

_____

_____

I'm Thankful for: _____

_____

_____

_____

_____

_____

Day Twenty-Four

"So then, those who suffer according to God's will should commit themselves to their faithful Creator and continue to do good."

1 Peter 4:19

Positive Reflection: _____

_____

_____

_____

_____

_____

Releasing Negativity: _____

_____

_____

_____

_____

_____

"Health is not valued
till sickness comes."

Thomas Fuller

Words of Encouragement: ————————————————

———————————————————————————————

———————————————————————————————

———————————————————————————————

———————————————————————————————

———————————————————————————————

I'm Thankful for: ————————————————————

———————————————————————————————

———————————————————————————————

———————————————————————————————

———————————————————————————————

———————————————————————————————

Day Twenty-Five

"My message and my preaching were not with wise and persuasive words, but with a demonstration of the Spirit's power, so that your faith might not rest on human wisdom, but on God's power."

1 Corinthians 2:4-5

Positive Reflection: _____

_____

_____

_____

_____

_____

Releasing Negativity: _____

_____

_____

_____

_____

_____

"Happiness is nothing more than good health and a bad memory."

Albert Schweitzer

Words of Encouragement: _____
_____
_____
_____
_____
_____

I'm Thankful for: _____
_____
_____
_____
_____
_____

Day Twenty-Six

"Finally, brethren, whatsoever things are true, whatsoever things are honest, whatsoever things are just, whatsoever things are pure, whatsoever things are lovely, whatsoever things are of good report: if there be any virtue, and if there be any praise, think on these things."

Philippians 4:8

Positive Reflection: _____

_____

_____

_____

_____

_____

Releasing Negativity: _____

_____

_____

_____

_____

_____

"My trust in God flows out of the experience of his loving me, day in and day out, whether the day is stormy or fair, whether I'm sick or in good health, whether I'm in a state of grace or disgrace. He comes to me where I live and loves me as I am."
Brennan Manning

Words of Encouragement: _____

_____

_____

_____

_____

_____

I'm Thankful for: _____

_____

_____

_____

_____

_____

Day Twenty-Seven

"...Be strong and courageous. Do not fear or be in dread of them, for it is the lord your God who goes with you. He will not leave you or forsake you."

Deuteronomy 31:6

Positive Reflection: _____

_____

_____

_____

_____

_____

Releasing Negativity: _____

_____

_____

_____

_____

_____

"A healthy attitude is contagious but don't wait to catch it from others. Be a carrier."

Tom Stoppard

Words of Encouragement: _____

_____

_____

_____

_____

_____

I'm Thankful for: _____

_____

_____

_____

_____

_____

Day Twenty-Eight

"On the day I called, you answered me;
my strength of soul you increased."

Psalms 138:3

Positive Reflection: _____
_____
_____
_____
_____
_____

Releasing Negativity: _____
_____
_____
_____
_____
_____

"Health is the thing
that makes you feel
that now is the best
time of the year."
Franklin Pierce Adams

Words of Encouragement: _____
_____
_____
_____
_____
_____

I'm Thankful for: _____
_____
_____
_____
_____
_____
_____

Day Twenty-Nine

"Come to me, all who labor and are heavy laden,
and I will give you rest. Take my yoke upon you,
and learn from me, for I am gentle and lowly in
heart, and you will find rest for your souls."

Matthew 11:28-29

Positive Reflection: _____

_____

_____

_____

_____

_____

Releasing Negativity: _____

_____

_____

_____

_____

_____

"Everybody needs beauty
as well as bread, places to
play in and pray in, where
nature may heal and give
strength to body and soul."
John Muir

Words of Encouragement: _____

_____

_____

_____

_____

_____

I'm Thankful for: _____

_____

_____

_____

_____

_____

Day Thirty

"Blessed be the God and Father of our lord Jesus Christ,
the Father of mercies and God of all comfort, who comforts
us in all our affliction, so that we may be able to comfort
those who are in any affliction, with the comfort with
which we ourselves are comforted by God."

2 Corinthians 1:3-4

Positive Reflection: _____

_____

_____

_____

_____

_____

Releasing Negativity: _____

_____

_____

_____

_____

_____

"Treasure the love you re-
ceive above all. It will sur-
vive long after your good
health has vanished."
Og Mandino

Words of Encouragement: _____

_____

_____

_____

_____

_____

_____

I'm Thankful for: _____

_____

_____

_____

_____

_____

_____

Day Thirty-One

"Our soul waits for the LORD; he is our help and our shield. For our heart is glad in him, because we trust in his holy name. Let your steadfast love, O LORD, be upon us, even as we hope in you."

Psalms 33:20-22

Positive Reflection: _____

_____

_____

_____

_____

_____

Releasing Negativity: _____

_____

_____

_____

_____

_____

"A person whose mind is quiet and satisfied in God is in the pathway to health."

Ellen G. White

Words of Encouragement: _____

_____

_____

_____

_____

_____

_____

I'm Thankful for: _____

_____

_____

_____

_____

_____

_____

My Blessings & Prayers

My prayer for you, and your loved ones!

The Lord said to Moses, "Tell Aaron and his sons, 'This is how you are to bless the Israelites. Say to them:

"The Lord bless you and keep you; the Lord make his face shine on you and be gracious to you; the Lord turn his face toward you and give you peace."

"So they will put my name on the Israelites, and I will bless them."

Numbers 6:22-27

With Much Joy,

Dellie Freeman

Made in the USA
Coppell, TX
15 May 2020

25572142R00043